ALZHEIMER'S DISEASE:

Home Care Planning and Management

Solomon Barroa, R.N.

Copyright 2012

All rights reserved. No part of this book may be reproduced by any means, electronic, mechanical, photocopying, recording, scanning or otherwise without permission from the author. The author reserves the right not to be responsible for the correctness, completeness or quality of the information provided. Liability claims regarding damage caused by the use of any information provided, including any kind of information that is incomplete or incorrect, will be rejected. The information contained in this book does not constitute medical advice, and is for information and educational purposes only. Consult your health care provider regarding health concerns.

To Dr. Lee Robbins, Mary Ann, Rosario, Vicente, Benedicto, and Robert.

PURPOSE:

The intention of this book is to educate the layperson and care providers about Alzheimer's disease and support her or him in moving towards a more effective role in managing the condition. This includes the many important interactions with medical professionals as well as other providers in the vast industry of diagnosis, services, supplements and information for Alzheimer's disease.

On the other hand, it is also my intention to provide readily accessible and useful information for medical professionals and other helping individuals such as family members, to support them effectively interacting with and assisting individuals with Alzheimer's disease or at risk for this condition.

In order to do so, this book provides substantial technical information about the body, its normal functions and how they are affected by Alzheimer's disease, the symptomatology and considerable practical advice regarding treatment and home care management. Some individuals reading the book will want to pursue all of these areas with equal intensity; others may find their needs focus more heavily on the nature of the disease itself or how to manage it. The Introduction and Table of Contents will assist readers in choosing whether to read the material from cover to cover or to focus upon particular issues covered in the various chapters. The Searchable nature of e-books will also assist readers to look up a particular topic of interest or importance to them. The reader should feel free to choose the sections of the text of greatest relevance and usefulness to you.

It is my intent as an author to be helpful to all readers and to encourage them to use this wide-ranging material in the manner that most strongly meets their needs. However, this book is not intended to constitute medical advice. The reader has the responsibility to consult a healthcare provider. The author welcomes your comments and suggestions and can be reached at:

solomon_barroa@yahoo.com

or at

http://www.amazon.com/Solomon-Barroa-RN/e/B00AV3V34S /

PLEASE SEE THE DOCTOR TO DISCUSS HEALTH CONCERNS. DON'T USE THIS TEXT FOR MEDICAL ADVICE OR DIAGNOSIS.

READING BEYOND THIS NOTICE IMPLIES YOU'VE READ AND AGREE TO THE ABOVE DISCLAIMER FOR YOUR OWN SAFETY. THANK YOU.

Introduction

The existence of different types of diseases across the globe has made humans very dependent on hospitalization and home care. The modernization of the healthcare system has helped prolong the life of a disease stricken person. State of the art technologies have shortened the span of the disease process.

One of the newer techniques in healthcare delivery is home care and outpatient treatment. The process of outpatient treatment has been an option for some conditions such as cataract extraction and minor wound care. However, there are certain diseases and illnesses that cannot be treated on an outpatient basis. Chronic diseases require long-term care and it is usually home based. Rising healthcare costs and limitations in covering healthcare services make it more difficult to effectively implement home healthcare. There are also certain diseases that are not curable and the cause is unknown. One of these is Alzheimer's disease.

Chapter 1 of this book gives the reader an introduction to Alzheimer's disease. Readers will get to know who discovered it, the definition of the disease, and its classification under the DSM IV TR (Diagnostic and Statistical Manual for Mental Disorders Text Revision).

Chapter 2 talks about possible causes and the mechanism behind Alzheimer's disease. There is no known, definitive cause of Alzheimer's disease. The possible causes presented in this book are still being investigated. We also discuss abnormal changes in the brain of the diagnosed person, such as the formation of tangles and plaques. The disease mechanism is commonly known in medical terms as the pathophysiology of the disease.

Chapter 3 is about the stages and symptoms of this disease. Each stage of the disease has varying degrees in terms of the severity of the symptoms. Symptoms are exemplified according to the stages of the disease.

Chapter 4 discusses the process of diagnosing and gathering evidence to confirm Alzheimer's disease is occurring in a person. Data gathering is the crucial step in formulating a diagnosis. This chapter covers general assessment, brain imaging, mental tests, neurological examination and laboratory tests, including a concise explanation of each procedure.

Chapter 5 concerns managing safety at home. Safety is a big concern, especially when family members are not around. For example, one must remove sharp pointed object and install an alarm system to help prevent falls inside the home.

Chapter 6 discusses management of different bodily symptoms using prescribed medications. Bodily symptoms that are manifested by a person with Alzheimer's disease are directly related to the affected area of the brain. There are memory problems, language impairment, incompetent judgment and behavioral symptoms. The medications such as cholinesterase inhibitors, antidepressants, anti-anxiety and neuroleptics are explained .

Chapter 7 talks about managing behavioral symptoms. The different types of behavioral symptoms are wandering, shadowing, sundowning, rummaging, pillaging, hoarding, agitation, aggression, hallucination, and delusion. This chapter provides the reader tips on how to handle and manage these symptoms.

Chapter 8 discusses communication techniques. Effective communication is the one of the hardest tasks in home care. Frequently, there is language impairment on the part of the diagnosed person. Techniques such as using simple sentences, acknowledging feelings, removing environmental noise and other means to ensure effective communication is discussed.

Chapter 9 describes managing the activities of daily living (ADL). ADLs include walking, bathing, dressing, eating and toileting. Frequently, these activities are not performed by the person undergoing the late stages of Alzheimer's disease. This imposes many burdens to caregivers and family members. This chapter provides important tips for managing ADLs.

Chapter 10, the final chapter, talks about basic home care management. Planning, organizing and intervening are the basic steps in management. Managing the home care needs to be flexible but directed toward achieving goals. This chapter identifies planning sets of actions, organizing to involve the diagnosed person and family members, and implementation to produce the desired results. We offer examples on preparing advance directives, managing safety at home, health insurance coverage, caregiver scheduling and bill payments.

Table of Contents

Chapter 1 — Defining and Classifying Alzheimer's Disease — 9

The Discovery of Alzheimer's Disease — 9
Defining Alzheimer's Disease — 9
Classifying Alzheimer's Disease — 10

Chapter 2 — Possible Causes and the Mechanism of Alzheimer's Disease — 11

Possible Causes of Alzheimer's Disease — 11
Mechanism of Alzheimer's Disease — 11
Tangles and Plaques on the Lobes of the Brain — 12

Chapter 3 — Stages and Symptoms of Alzheimer's Disease — 14

Stage 1 Absent to Pre-mild Impairment in Cognition — 14
Stage 2 Mild to Pre-moderate Impairment in Cognition — 14
Stage 3 Moderate to Pre-severe Impairment in Cognition — 14
Stage 4 Severe Impairment in Cognition — 15
Stage 5 Absence of Competent Cognition / Late stage — 15

Chapter 4 — Diagnosing Alzheimer's Disease — 16

General Assessment and Medical History of the Person with Alzheimer's Disease — 16
Brain Imaging — 17
Evaluating the Mental Status through a Test — 17
Neurological Examination — 18
Laboratory Tests — 18

Chapter 5 — Managing the Safety of a Person with Alzheimer's Disease — 19

Removal of Objects that Can Cause Physical Injuries — 19
Blocking and Guarding Power Sources — 19
Preventing Fall Accidents — 20
Installing Devices to Prevent Leaving the House — 20

Chapter 6 — Managing the Care of Bodily Symptoms through Prescribed Medications — 21

Administering Drugs for the Brain — 21
Administering Drugs to Manage Secondary Symptoms — 22
A. Administering Antidepressants — 22
B. Administering Anxiolytics — 22
C. Administering Neuroleptics — 22

Chapter 7 — Managing and Intervening the Behavioral Symptoms   24

The Shadowing Behavior   *24*
The Wandering Behavior   *24*
The Sundowning Behavior   *25*
The Rummaging, Hoarding and Pillaging Behavior   *25*
The Agitated and Aggressive Behavior   *25*
Behaviors Resulting From Hallucination and Delusions   *26*
Managing Disturbances in Self Concept   *27*

Chapter 8 — Effectively Communicating to a Person with the Alzheimer's Disease   28

Techniques of Communicating With the Diagnosed Person   *28*

Chapter 9 — Managing the Activities of Daily Living   29

Managing Eating   *29*
Managing Bathing and Personal Hygiene   *29*
Managing Toilet and Elimination   *30*
Managing Dressing   *30*
Managing Ambulation and Walking   *31*
Managing Activities   *31*

Chapter 10 — Basic Home Care Management   32

References   34

Index   35

Chapter 1 — Defining and Classifying Alzheimer's Disease

Who discovered Alzheimer's disease? Normally, discoveries and inventions are named after the person who discovered it. The person who discovered the Alzheimer's disease is a doctor by the name of Aloysius Alzheimer. His background is neuropathology and he is known to use silver staining technique.

Traditionally, we have known that doctors are the primary care providers for any patient in a hospital setting. They perform a thorough assessment, formulate a diagnosis, plan the treatment method, implement it and evaluate the outcome. There are instances when the presenting symptoms are uncommon and extraordinary to the broad knowledge of a doctor. All possible treatments necessary to alleviate the prevailing symptoms are performed. Misdiagnosis can happen at times, leading to a second opinion or the death of the sickened person. If death occurs and the doctor is unsure about the disease, an autopsy may be performed to investigate.

The Discovery of Alzheimer's Disease

In 1901, a German doctor by the name of Aloysius Alzheimer noticed unusual symptoms from one of his middle aged female patients. The symptoms were memory loss and bizarre cognition attributed to disorientation in time and place. He consulted some of his colleagues about the symptoms but it wasn't clear what caused them. Years passed and Dr. Alzheimer had not treated the unusual symptoms of his female patient. Finally, in 1906, the female patient died. After the death of his patient, he used silver stain to the brain of the patient to investigate and understand what really happened inside the brain. He found there were plaques and tangles in the brain. He then presented his findings adding the possibility of pre senile dementia. Pre senile dementia is a kind of dementia that can happen to a person before reaching the age of senility.

Defining Alzheimer's Disease

Alzheimer's disease is defined as a progressive disorder of cognitive abilities that fall under one of the categories of dementia. A dementia is a disorder that affects the brain and produces a set of symptoms or a syndrome. The symptoms are memory loss, problems with language, inability to do problem solving, and disorientation to time, places, and persons. The most common types of dementia are Alzheimer's type, vascular related dementias and those with Lewy bodies in the brain. The Alzheimer type of dementia has the presence of abnormal structures such as tangles and plaques inside the brain causing the display of symptoms. Vascular dementia, otherwise known as multi infarct dementia, is a disruption in the flow of oxygenated blood to the brain. It is usually caused by a blockage to the blood vessels such as those in people who suffered from stroke. The Lewy body type of dementia, discovered by Friedrich Lewy, has round like structures inside the brain known as lewy bodies, causing cognitive disabilities.

Classifying Alzheimer's Disease

Classifying Alzheimer's disease has been controversial over the years. At the present time, it is classified as a mental disorder. One way of classifying a mental disorder is that it should have a definitive diagnosis under the DSM IV (Diagnostic and Statistical Manual of Mental Disorders). The DSM is a manual that guides mental health professional in diagnosing and categorizing mental disorders. The DSM has been revised and the current revision is the fourth one. Alzheimer's disease is currently classified as Axis 3 in the Diagnostic and Statistical Manual of Mental Disorders (DSM IV). It falls under Dementia of the Alzheimer's Type as either early onset or late onset. The early onset type of dementia occurs before the age of 60 whereas late onset occurs after the age of 60. The code that is used is 331.0 to mean Alzheimer's disease, however code 290 is used to differentiate symptoms associated with the early and late onset types. According to the DSM, dementia of the Alzheimer's type either the early or late onset has associated symptoms. These symptoms could be uncomplicated, with delirium, with delusions or with a depressive mood. It is cautionary that only well trained mental health professionals such as a psychiatrist will classify a particular mental disorder. Through this process, more careful attention in terms of planning and intervention is implemented.

Chapter 2 — Possible Causes and the Mechanism of Alzheimer's Disease

Possible Causes of Alzheimer's Disease

The cause of Alzheimer's disease is unknown. The presence of tangles and plaques in the later stage of the disease causes more profound symptoms that are displayed by the person with the disease. Nonetheless, these tangles and plaques are being analyzed regarding what causes them to develop in the brain. Some of the causes that were suggested and under investigation are the roles of genes, inflammatory conditions of the brain, environmental factors, the aging process, dietary intake, lack of mental exercises and co morbidity or existence of another medical condition. Genes are transmitted from parents to offspring. Research findings showed the presence of the genes ApoE4 (apolipoprotein) existed in late stages of the Alzheimer's disease. Mutations of the genes PSI (presenilin) 1 and 2, and APP (amyloid precursor protein) are also believed to have caused the disease. Inflammatory condition of the brain produces elemental compounds causing the disease. Environmental exposure to greater amount of aluminum, pesticides and other types of toxins are also viewed as causative factors. The process of aging naturally exposes an individual to free radicals inside the body. There is continues wear and tear as free radicals develop in greater quantity imposing death to the brain cells. Intake of food with insufficient nutrients is also viewed as a causative factor particularly Vitamin E. Mental exercises such as social networking stimulates cognitive abilities. It promotes problem solving, interaction and intellectual stimulation. Certain studies showed that lack of mental exercises are prevalent in people with Alzheimer's disease. Finally, the existence of co morbid conditions in the body is viewed as a causative factor for the disease. Researchers are exploring the connection of the shingles virus to the formation of plaques and tangles. It is believed the shingles virus can cross the blood brain barrier and multiply in the brain. All of these causative factors have never been confirmed until now. Much research is being conducted to further understand the factors that cause Alzheimer's disease. The tangles and plaques can best be confirmed when the person dies and a postmortem evaluation or autopsy is performed.

Mechanism of Alzheimer's Disease

In order to understand the mechanism of the disease, a person has to understand the parts and functions of the central nervous system in the body. The central nervous system consists of three major parts: the brain, spinal cord and the neurons. Any defect in these three major parts will affect the integrity of the entire system.

The brain regulates the functionality of the different organs of the body. It processes memory, reasoning, judgment, language, emotions, sensation, orientation and other cognitive activities.

There are four lobes of the brain: the frontal, temporal, parietal, and occipital. The lobes of the brain are generally known as the cerebral cortex. Judgment, problem solving and other intellectual activities are processed in the frontal lobe. The parietal lobe processes the interpretation of sensation through the sense organs of the body. Visual interpretation is processed by the occipital lobe. The temporal lobe processes smell and sound stimulus. The main structure of the brain that makes human rational is the frontal lobe. The hippocampus is a part of the brain that is located above the brain stem. It is also called medial temporal lobe and sub cortical area of the brain. It functions to store memories.

Neurons are nerve cells that transmit and send information. There are two types of neurons, the sensory and motor. Sensory neurons transmit sensation from the sensory organs. Motor neurons send the signal coming from the brain to the body creating movement. The major parts of the neuron are axon, dendrite and the cell body. Axons and dendrites are filament like structures that is extended from the cell body. Axon sends signal to another neuron whereas dendrite receive signals from other neurons. A synapse is a connection between the axon and dendrite of two neurons, and this where signals are transmitted. Inside the neuron, there are cellular structures such as nucleus and microtubules. The microtubules guide the nutrients inside the neural cell and it is stabilized by a protein called tau. Neurons also release neurotransmitters to excite or inhibit a reaction such as acetylcholine. Neurons are always electrically charged causing either excitability or inhibition.

The spinal cord starts from the occipital bone and ends at the second lumbar vertebrae. It is contained inside the vertebral bones, which are segmented. The vertebral bones are seven in the cervical area, twelve in thoracic area, five in lumbar area, and one in coccyx and sacrum. Spinal nerves arise from the spinal cord. The spinal cord functions to transmit signals to and from the body and coordinate reflexes.

Tangles and Plaques on the Lobes of the Brain

Tangles occur inside the axon and dendrites of the neural cell. The tau protein, which stabilizes the microtubules inside the neural cell, undergoes changes through a chemical reaction. The chemical changes cause the tau protein to bind with another tau protein leading to a tangle like structure. When there is a tangle, it causes detachment and disintegration of the microtubules and it results to the impairment of the transmission of signals. It eventually leads to the death of the neural cells. The tangles are insoluble.

Plaques occur outside the cell membrane of the neural cell. The amyloid precursor protein, which is needed by the cell membrane of the neuron, adheres partly inside and outside of the cellular membrane. Enzymes act on these protein and split it up into fragmented parts. These fragmented parts are called beta amyloid. After a chemical reaction, these proteins clump together and join other non-cellular entities, forming an insoluble plaque.

Tangles and plaques occur primarily in the hippocampus and extend to the frontal lobe of the brain. The presence of these plaques and tangles on the hippocampus and frontal lobe impairs their functionality and in turn affects the entire integrity of the brain. Memory loss is the initial sign of Alzheimer's disease. This is due to the hippocampus being infiltrated by plaques and tangles. It eventually extends up to the cerebral cortex and the whole brain. The progression of the damage depends on factors such as the person's genetic makeup, lifestyle, diet and environmental hazards. There is no treatment and cure.

Chapter 3 — Stages and Symptoms of Alzheimer's Disease

A basic understanding of the stages and symptoms that go with the disease usually prepares caregivers and loved ones to manage the home care of the person with Alzheimer's disease. It is not necessary to have a medical background but one must have an open mind and accepting attitude to effectively manage care. The stages of Alzheimer's disease differ from one book to another and from one organization to another. We present the stages based upon the different materials that were used in writing this book.

Stage 1 Absent to Pre-mild Impairment in Cognition

Initially in this stage, there is no memory loss. The person with the disease is competent in all their cognitive abilities. It is hypothesized the disease may have started ten years earlier in the hippocampus of the brain. As tangles and plaques become greater in number, they then gradually elicit mild symptoms of memory loss such as forgetting the location of the key to the house or where eyeglasses were placed.

Stage 2 Mild to Pre-moderate Impairment in Cognition

The tangles and plaques have grown in numbers during this stage. All the symptoms in this stage have become noticeable to friends and members of the household. Planning and organizing daily activities has declined. The process of reading and comprehension produces minimal retention of important details about what was read. Frequently, there is misplacing and loss of previously handled objects such as a car key. There is an inability to recall and remember the names of persons that are introduced during a social activity. There are apparent problems in naming an object or thinking of a word to relate to an object in sight. There are instances where a judgment is made, such as buying an expensive handbag. The length of time to accomplish daily tasks and activities is getting longer than usual. There is some confusion about location of familiar places such as parks and grocery stores. Some mistakes are committed in computing finances and in paying house bills. There is also a change in personality and disturbances in mood.

Stage 3 Moderate to Pre-severe Impairment in Cognition

In this stage, the plaques and tangles has spread to areas of the cerebral cortex. This stage has profound effects on language abilities, reasoning skills, sensory processing and conscious thought. Symptoms are more evident and safety is compromised. Knowledge of recent events that occurred is significantly decreased. The memory of one's personal history is minimally recalled. Confusion about places, names of persons and dates is more profound. There is total inability to recall details about residential address, telephone numbers and other important personal information. The ability to learn new things is deficient. There is absence of coping abilities regarding new and unexpected situations. Significant loss of impulse control is profound, such that vulgar language and undressing at inappropriate times is common. There is wandering in the late afternoon and tearfulness at times. Perception and motor problems persist such that the person will have difficulty getting out of a chair. There is difficulty in thinking logically about situations and events. Movements and word statements are done in a repetitive fashion. There are psychological symptoms such as hallucinations, delusions about self and events, suspiciousness about persons and constant irritability. Profound difficulty in language, reading, writing and working with numbers is noticed by everybody. At this stage, the person is still able to retain information about his or her own name including the spouse and family members.

Stage 4 Severe Impairment in Cognition

The tangles and plaques are widespread on major areas of the brain. Awareness of recent events and experiences is mostly lost. There is still an ability to recall one's own name but not the personal history. Frequently, the patient forgets the name of the caregiver and family members. Assistance in performing activities of daily living such as dressing and toileting is constant. Increases occur in episodes of bowel and bladder incontinence. The normal circadian rhythm of sleeping and wakefulness is disrupted. There is constant wandering in places and getting lost more often. Psychological and behavioral symptoms such as hallucinations, delusions and suspicions are more profound. Repetitive behavior such as playing with tissue paper is a daily occurrence. There is clinical terminology that is used in relation to the observed symptoms such as agnosia or loss of ability to recognize and identify objects and persons, apraxia or inability to use objects, despite of knowledge on how to use them and aphasia or impairment in the ability to use language.

Stage 5 Absence of Competent Cognition / Late stage

This is the last stage of Alzheimer's disease wherein plaques and tangles are widespread all over the brain. Recognizing one's own family and friends does not exist anymore. There is no capacity for recognized speech and words don't mean anything. Performing self-care is impossible and there is total dependence on caregivers for survival. There is no bowel and bladder control. There is difficulty in swallowing any food or water causing weight loss. The ability to perform activities of daily living such as walking or sitting is lost. Frequent and constant moaning, groaning and grunting is evident in all instances. The sense about self and one's existence is gone. Death is imminent. Hospice care is an option for some family members especially if care is burdensome.

Chapter 4 — Diagnosing Alzheimer's Disease

Diagnosing a person with Alzheimer's disease requires an accurate assessment and a number of tests and procedures. This chapter will discuss the general assessment and the most common procedures a physician will order to confirm the diagnosis.

General Assessment and Medical History of the Person with Alzheimer's Disease

A history encompasses all the information and events that happened. Initially, the basic information about the identity of the person such as name, address, social security number, and insurance policy is gathered through an interview. Asking questions is a hurdle because of memory loss and language barriers for non-English speakers. A family member or a translator is necessary to gather accurate information.

A packet of questions can also be sent to the person to complete with the help of a household member, and then brought to the interview.

After gathering general information, a comprehensive review of current and past medical conditions is done. Hospitalizations, surgeries, previous and current diagnosis are some of the information that is asked. These will enable the nurse or physician to understand if co morbidity causes the symptoms of the disease.

All the prescribed and over the counter medications are listed and verified. Some drugs have synergistic actions and can lead to serious side effects that can mask some of the symptoms. It is also a means to check and verify if a medication is appropriately prescribed or not.

An assessment of the over all functionality is done to know if there has been limited performance in activities of daily living such as bathing, ambulating, toileting, eating, and dressing. The instrumental activities of daily living such as shopping, using the telephone, driving skills, and cooking are also asked. In the late stage of Alzheimer's disease, all of the activities of daily living are impaired or not performed at all.

A social and psychological history is then gathered. The person is asked about the family dynamics, occupation and leisure, marital status and if there are conflicts, spirituality and religion, social support, stress level and coping abilities, alcohol and recreational drug usage, feelings about self and the future, and if there are changes in the person's value system.

Finally, the home environment is assessed. It is best to visit the home of the person with Alzheimer's disease to have an accurate assessment. The bathroom is checked for accessibility, ease of use and if there are assistive devices. The stairs are checked for safety to prevent a fall episode. Smoke and carbon monoxide detectors, personal emergency response system, accessibility to emergency numbers, the presence of food and means of cooking them are also checked. Environmental hazards and fall risk factors are immediately identified and discussed with the person together with the household members or caregivers.

Brain Imaging

The process of creating images from the brain can be done trough an MRI (magnetic resonance imaging), CT (computed tomography), and PET (positron emission tomography) scan. In a CT scan, a contrast or dye (iodine based) is usually injected into the veins. The person lies on a narrow bed and the head is then advanced under a CT scanner where there is an X-ray tube and detector to capture images of the brain. Exposure to radiation is usually minimal but higher in doses. There are also people who are allergic to the contrast that is to be injected to the vein. Informing the physician regarding allergy to iodine is important to prevent allergic reaction, which can be fatal. For an MRI scan, the injection of a contrast may be done in some cases. The person lies on the examination table and the head is then enclosed under a cylinder that will capture the images. In a PET scan, a radioactive tracer is injected through an intravenous line in the arm. The person lies on a table and entered through the PET machine where images are captured. Instructions about doing some cognitive abilities such as computing mathematical operations or chronological orders of words may be asked to ascertain functionality of the brain. PET scans are usually expensive and seldom ordered. All of these scans require the person to remain still while the process is taking place. Care should be taken when standing after the procedure to prevent falls due to dizziness and possible orthostatic hypotension (drop in blood pressure). There is also an order to empty the bladder and prevent excessive fluid intake prior to the procedure and to maintain adequate hydration after the procedure.

Evaluating the Mental Status through a Test

There are a number of mental tests that can be used to assess the mental status of the person with Alzheimer's disease. The most commonly used is the MMSE (Mini Mental State Examination). The MMSE, also known as Folstein test, is used to screen functionality regarding orientation to time and place, registering names of objects, calculation and attention to numbers and words, recalling what was registered in the memory, language competence through identifying objects, repetition skills by repeating a phrase, ability to carry out complex commands such as instructions to fold a paper and put it on the floor, obeying a command to close the eyes, write a sentence, and draw and copy a particular shape. The person is also asked to answer questions regarding judgment and reasoning, questions such as why taking somebody else's medication is harmful and what to do during a fire. The objective of MMSE is to assess functionality in areas of memory and recall, simple arithmetic, language and comprehension, orientation to time and place and psychomotor skills in carrying out simple tasks. Language barriers, sensory deficits, and educational attainment are factors that need to be considered before interpreting the MMSE.

Neurological Examination

A neurological examination is performed to determine other bodily conditions that can cause the signs and symptoms of the person with Alzheimer's disease such as Parkinson's disease. It comprises of a set of interview questions and a physical examination of the nervous system. The physical aspect of the neurological examination measures the responsiveness of the cerebellum, the ability to interpret sensation, the presence of deep tendon reflexes, the competence of the motor system of the body, and the reactivity of the cranial nerves. The cerebellum is a part of the brain that regulates motor movement of the body and some cognitive activities related to attention and language. Cranial nerves are twelve pairs of nerves that arise from the brain which functions for sensory and motor sensations. These cranial nerves are olfactory (smelling), optic (vision), oculomotor (upper eyelid and eyeball movement), trochlear (eyeball movement), trigeminal (mastication and facial sensation), abducens (eye ball movement), facial (facial expression), vestibulocochlear (sense of balance and hearing), glossopharyngeal (taste), vagus (muscles of larynx and pharynx), accessory (head and shoulder movement), and hypoglossal (swallowing and tongue movement). Mental status tests are also a part of the total neurological examination.

Laboratory Tests

The main objective of laboratory tests is to determine if there is a co morbid condition causing the symptoms that are presented by the person with Alzheimer's disease. These laboratory tests are mandatory assisting with the accuracy of the diagnosis. Laboratory tests that will be ordered are actually blood tests. The laboratory tests that are ordered by the physician are complete blood count, blood chemistry work which focuses on the different electrolytes or chemical elements in the blood, analysis of the urine, studies about the function of the liver, hormone levels specifically with the thyroid stimulating hormone, levels of vitamin B12 and folate, and tests to detect the presence of bacteria and viruses such as in syphilis and HIV.

The final and definitive diagnosis of Alzheimer's disease requires a lot of work, effort and a considerable period of time. It is very costly as well. The existence of a health care insurance is important during this entire process.

Chapter 5 — Managing the Safety of a Person with Alzheimer's Disease

After the diagnosis of Alzheimer's disease, there are numerous issues that confront the family and love ones of the person with Alzheimer's disease such as telling the diagnosed person about his or her diagnosis, the living will and durable power of attorney, the person that will act as the caregiver, the expenses that will incur regarding medicine and medical services, and among many other issues. Guidance and counseling is beneficial for the loved ones of the diagnosed person. The location for the care is to be decided. Home care is less expensive when compared to an Alzheimer's unit in a facility. The ability to monitor the safety of the person with Alzheimer's disease is comforting to loved ones, though there is more technology and time allotment that is used in an Alzheimer's facility. Stage three and four of the Alzheimer's disease requires constant care and personal safety is considered to be the one of the biggest concerns.

The impact of the cognitive impairment to the bodily process needs to be understood in planning and managing for the safety of the diagnosed person. The normal process of aging also implies safety issues. There is sensory and perceptual alteration that decreases the ability of the diagnosed person to react to certain stimuli at home, such as the smell of smoke from a fire, the ringing of a doorbell and different signs that are posted in the house. Bodily changes in relation to the muscles and nervous system may render the diseased person to fall frequently. The inability to rationalize causes and effects of certain actions greatly affect safety. The absence of impulse control can lead to overmedication and accidental intake of harmful chemicals. Usage of knife and cutting instruments may produce skin wounds. Aspiration is a risk due to difficulty in swallowing food.

Removal of Objects that Can Cause Physical Injuries

The initial plan when managing safety at home is to remove all objects that can cause bodily harm such as knives and sharp pointed objects, chemically concentrated products such as insecticides and cleaning fluids, anything that is fragile or can be broken, aerosol and paint cans, appliances including flat irons, power tools that are used for construction and medications that are usually overdosed by the cognitively impaired person.

Blocking and Guarding Power Sources

Inappropriate use of electrical outlets produces burns. The impaired cognition of the diagnosed person will not recognize the danger of electrical current. Blocking or guarding stove knobs prevents misuse that can cause accidental burns. The thermostat needs to be guarded as well because the diagnosed person is incompetent in sensing changes in room temperature, as that may either lead to hyperthermia or hypothermia as consequences of extremes in temperature.

Preventing Fall Accidents

Falling is a threat to older adults at all times. The risk is doubled when there is cognitive impairment. Always maintain clear pathways. Passageways such as the hall should be well lighted especially at nighttime. One should remove all cords that are extended as well as throw rugs around the house, and make sure that stair railings are secure and attached well. The diagnosed person should use non-skid shoes and not use furniture with wheels.

Installing Devices to Prevent Leaving the House

Wandering behavior is constant in 3rd and 4th stages of the disease. Use double locks to all doors and windows that can be used as an exit route, install warning devices and buzzers on doors to detect if the diagnosed person is trying to leave, place wrist bands which can trigger alarm to signal if the person attempted to leave the house, and install a monitoring system that can be accessed in a television or a computer.

Chapter 6 — Managing the Care of Bodily Symptoms through Prescribed Medications

Bodily symptoms from the person diagnosed with Alzheimer's disease are directly related to impaired cognitive abilities. As plaques and tangles increase in numbers and continuously destroy parts of the brain, signs and symptoms of the disease become more profound. The physician will prescribe different drugs that will manage the symptoms manifested by the diagnosed person. There is no cure for Alzheimer's disease but, rather, symptoms are treated with different kinds of drugs.

People with the Alzheimer's disease are unable to prepare their own medications. They will forget the daily schedule and not understand the importance of dosages. In fact, their tendency is to overmedicate. A member of the household or a caregiver should prepare these medications in pill boxes and constantly remind the diseased person about it. Dosage and scheduling is done by the physician. Compliance to the medication regimen is a must.

Administering Drugs for the Brain

The drugs that will enable cognitive functionality of the diseased person are called ChEIs (Cholinesterase inhibitors), aimed at preventing the breakdown of the neurotransmitter acetylcholine. The neurotransmitter acetylcholine functions as a neuron modulator and forms the cholinergic system with neurons in the central nervous system. There are at least four known ChEIs, namely: Donepizil (Aricept), Rivastigmine (Exelon), Galantamine (Razadyne) and Tacrine. Aricept is usually prescribed at 5-10 mg once daily for mild to moderate stages of the disease and 10-25 mg once daily for moderate to severe stages of the disease. Exelon is prescribed at least 1.5 mg twice daily for mild to moderate stages of the disease. Razadyne is usually prescribed at 4 mg twice daily for mild to moderate stages of the disease. Tacrine is not prescribed anymore because it is toxic to the liver. The common side effects of ChEIs are gastrointestinal discomfort such as nausea, vomiting and diarrhea. It also causes dizziness and fainting, which predisposes the diseased person to fall accidents. An understanding about side effects of these drugs will prepare the caregiver and household members about necessary intervention, care and safety measures.

For moderate to severe stages of the disease, another drug option can be prescribed. This drug is called Memantine (Namenda) and it is an antagonist for NMDA (N Methyl D Aspartate). The NMDA is a kind of a glutamate receptor that helps in memory and learning, and it destroys nerve cells if the amount is excessively high. Namenda blocks the NMDA glutamate receptors to prevent further damage. The common side effects are drowsiness, dizziness, confusion at times, mild headache, inability to sleep and some degree of agitation. Constant monitoring and supervision is needed to prevent falls due to drowsiness and dizziness. Reorientation is also done because of confusion and agitation.

Administering Drugs to Manage Secondary Symptoms

A. Administering Antidepressants

Depression and mood changes occur as secondary symptoms primarily because the parts of the brain are infiltrated with tangles and plaques. There is impairment in processing emotions and the mood throughout the day. Antidepressants are drugs used to treat symptoms of depression because they block the reuptake of certain neurotransmitters such as serotonin and norepinephrine. There are many classes of antidepressant that can be used such as the tricyclic antidepressant (TCA), monoamine oxidase inhibitor (MAOI) and selective serotonin reuptake inhibitor (SSRI). The most commonly used antidepressants are Amitriptyline (Elavil), Bupropion (Wellbutrin), Mirtazapine (Remeron), Duloxetine (Cymbalta), Citalopram (Celexa), Fluoxetine (Prozac), Escitalopram (Lexapro) and Sertraline (Zoloft). Dry mouth, drowsiness, insomnia and some gastrointestinal disturbances such as nausea are common side effects of these drugs. Assistance and monitoring should be implemented on a daily basis. It is always prudent to research and ask the physician about these drugs. Dosage and frequency may be altered depending on the degree of depression and mood changes.

B. Administering Anxiolytics

Persons with Alzheimer's disease are often anxious and agitated. This is primarily because feelings and emotions are incompetently processed in the brain. There are prescribed medication under the category of anxiolytic (anti anxiety) that are used to treat anxiety and agitation. Majority of anxiolytic medications belong to the class of benzodiazepines. The most commonly prescribed anti-anxiety medications are Lorazepam (Ativan), Diazepam (Valium), Clonazepam (Klonopin) and Chlordiaxepoxide (Librium). The common side effects are dry mouth, drowsiness, lightheadedness and some confusion. Supervision, assistance and monitoring is of the essence when taking these drugs. Always ask the physician regarding the side effects. Dosage and frequency of these drugs will be dependent on the severity of the symptom presented.

C. Administering Neuroleptics

There is hallucination and delusion at the severe and late stages of the Alzheimer's disease. These symptoms are managed through the administration of neuroleptics that acts to decrease its occurrence. Neuroleptics are antipsychotic drugs that stop the uptake of dopamine that causes the psychotic episodes. The most commonly used neuroleptics are Risperidone (Risperdal), Olanzapine (Zyprexa), Quetiapine (Seroquel), Thioridazine (Mellaril), Chlorpromazine (Thorazine), Promethazine (Phenergan) and Prochlorperazine (Compazine). There are common side effects when taking these drugs such as tardive dyskinesia or involuntary repetitive movement, akathisia or inability to stay still, agranulocytosis or lowered white blood cell count, rigidity and tremors. It definitely requires constant monitoring, supervision and assistance on a daily basis.

The side effects from any of these prescribed drugs will vary from one person to another. Some people will not experience any side effects at all but some might go beyond the common side effects. Sudden withdrawal from taking these drugs will produce untoward bodily reactions such that side effects will worsen. Tapering these medications to lower doses will enable the body to gradually adjust to the process of withdrawal.

Chapter 7 — Managing and Intervening the Behavioral Symptoms

The person with Alzheimer's disease has basic needs just like anybody else. Some of these needs are biological such as food, rest, elimination and exercises. If these needs are not met, it leads to agitation, combativeness, withdrawal, refusing to participate in self-care, anxiety and other behavioral problems. Daily assessment and observation regarding signs of infection, dehydration, incontinence and blood sugar imbalance also prompts both the caregiver and household members to intervene and inform the physician. Any co morbid or co existing conditions that may arise or that are acquired from the disease will result in behavioral symptoms and complications.

The Shadowing Behavior

Shadowing is a terminology to mean that the diagnosed person follows the caregiver or any household member around the house and may ask a lot of questions. This kind of behavior can be tiresome and annoying. To manage this behavior, assess if there is a trigger factor such as a child that prompts the shadowing. Removing or adjusting the trigger factor often stops the shadowing behavior. If there aren't any noticeable trigger factors, distraction and preoccupation with an activity such as chewing a candy or helping to remove dust from furniture is a good intervention.

The Wandering Behavior

Wandering means a process of walking that seem to appear as aimless but often has a purpose for the wanderer. It can be a way for coping with stressful situation around the house or it could be that the wanderer is looking for something and someone. There are at least two types of wandering behavior, the purposeful and none purposeful. The purposeful wandering behavior occurs in a routine fashion and it is usually a means to escape from boredom or to do some exercises. It is predictable and happens at the same time of each day at the same place. None purposeful type of wandering is aimless and the wanderer enters somebody's room or take another person's belonging. There is also an escapist type of wandering behavior that is purposeful because the wanderer has a destination to go somewhere or meet someone.

There are ways to manage a wandering behavior such as providing a safe environment to walk without incidental falls by removing clutter and throw rugs, installing locks and alarm systems, putting identification bracelet with name and address, remove objects that will stimulate wandering such as purses and coats. If the wandering person has left the house in a distance, approach him or her from the front then calmly redirect by walking alongside and gradually maneuver them back to the house. The schedule of wandering behavior should be noted and listed in a journal so that interventions can be easily implemented.

The Sundowning Behavior

The sundowning behavior means a restless behavior sometime during night or evening hours. It could be due to fatigue, bodily discomfort, loneliness, disturbing dreams, perceive shadows from bedroom lights, side effects of medication or from caffeinated drinks. This behavior can be managed by maintaining good sleep hygiene with regular night time routine, avoiding stimulants such as coffee or noises before bedtime, administering pain relievers, placing a bedside commode, closing window blinds to avoid shadows and evaluating prescribed medication and their side effects. The sundowning behavior can be exhausting to caregivers and members of the household as it disrupts their sleep and can cause an accident on the part of the diagnosed person. Addressing the cause of the behavior will prevent its timely occurrence.

The Rummaging, Hoarding and Pillaging Behavior

Rummaging behavior implies searching for something in a pile of clothes or other objects. Hoarding behavior means accumulating objects that was gathered from another place. Pillaging behavior means taking an object that is owned by another person. These three behaviors are combined automatically as a routine for a person with Alzheimer's disease. It is believed that the behavior is intended to search and take an object of value. The objects that were taken are usually of the same significance and of the same type. This type of behavior results in clutters and missing or misplaced objects. Managing this behavior can be done by placing stock supplies in a locked place, keeping personal belongings in a secure place, locking or closing bedroom doors at all times and returning objects to their previous locations to prevent hoarding. It is not advisable to confront the diagnosed person or to get hysterical about this behavior. Caregivers and household members need to evaluate the objects that were taken and analyze its importance to the diseased person. Through this analysis, a creative plan such as an activity can be implemented to involve the person and redirect this behavior. An example would be creating a file of folders if the person is pillaging and hoarding about folders and papers.

The Agitated and Aggressive Behavior

An agitated behavior is an emotional state of excitement and restlessness that is either manifested in physical or verbal means. The common causes of agitation in a person with Alzheimer's disease are needs that are not met, bodily discomfort, environmental factors, effects of medication and confusion. An aggressive behavior is a hostile tendency toward self, other people or an object. There is an intention to cause harm or to dominate a particular situation. Aggression is most often caused by agitation. Managing agitation and aggression can be very difficult to caregivers and members of the household. The initial thing to do is to assess and identify the causes or the trigger factor. Removing the cause or the trigger usually works for most people.

Approach the agitated person calmly and in a gentle tone. Avoid confrontation, reasoning and lengthy explanations. Do not force the agitated person to do something that they do not want to do because it will result in aggressive behavior. If the agitated person is resistant, distraction and diversion may be an option. Try to move the agitated person to a quiet place. A gentle touch is often therapeutic. Always speak in a soothing voice and avoid being authoritative.

Behaviors Resulting From Hallucination and Delusions

A delusion is defined as a false belief that is strongly upheld despite contrary to factual evidence. The most common delusions are grandiosity, persecution, and of a specific theme. Delusion of grandeur is a belief that someone has special powers, abilities, skills or fame. The delusion of persecution is a belief that someone is being poisoned, followed or there is a conspiracy against him or her. Delusions that are of specific themes include somatic, guilt, religion, reference and control.

Hallucination is defined as a perception in the absence of a real stimulus. It is distorted and unreal because of the absence of factual basis. The most common hallucinations are that of vision, auditory, somatic and olfactory. Visual hallucinations exemplify seeing flashes of light or objects. Hearing voices or sounds of animals is an example of auditory hallucination. Somatic hallucinations exemplify bodily mutilation or disembowelment. Smelling fecal matter or urine is an example of olfactory hallucination.

Delusions and hallucinations are regarded as psychotic symptoms. For a person with Alzheimer's disease these symptoms can be a result of medication, bodily condition, stress and emotional insecurity. If these symptoms are not handled appropriately, it may lead to aggressive tendencies, fearsome attitude and violence. Consulting a psychiatrist or a trained mental health professional is essential.

Managing hallucination and delusions is one of the hardest tasks to do. An effective communication system, monitoring schedule and teamwork is needed. Avoid arguing or disagreeing with the diagnosed person regarding what they perceived or sensed. It usually leads to agitation and violence. Scan and check the environment for trigger factors such as noises that was misinterpreted. Analyze or consider if delusions and hallucinations are based on the person's past history. Remove the trigger factor such as a mirror that can be misinterpreted as an image of another person. Use distraction such as playing music or taking the diagnosed person to the garden.

Medications are usually prescribed by the physician if any or all of the above behaviors are impossible to handle. Managing these behaviors require teamwork. Caregivers and household members are the people who confront it everyday. The assessment about the severity of the symptoms and the trigger factor is needed by the physician and the members of the healthcare team to plan and implement a new set of action.

Managing Disturbances in Self Concept

The concept of one's self is greatly impaired during the disease process resulting in low self-esteem and feelings of hopelessness. Reminiscing is a therapy that can restore this. It may not be applicable during the last stages of the disease. It is believed that reminiscing is an effective therapy because long-term memory remains intact for a long time. Life review is a type of reminiscing. The diagnosed person recalls past experiences. It reevaluates the past in order to settle and integrate what was in conflict back then. Reminiscing the most significant events promotes a sense of accomplishment. It also gives a sense of pride that raises self esteem.

Chapter 8 — Effectively Communicating to a Person with the Alzheimer's Disease

Communication is a process of sending and receiving information through verbal and non-verbal means. Verbal communication is executed through speaking or talking, and non-verbal communication occurs through writing, bodily gestures and expression. The basic element of the communication process is the existence of a sender, a message and a receiver. A person with Alzheimer's disease has an impaired communication process. The left area of the brain regulates language, reasoning and calculation. Aphasia is a common occurrence. It involves language impairment in speaking, reading, writing and calculating.

There is difficulty in word association and word finding during the first stage, exemplified by using the word truck instead of car. There is also repetition of what was said because of forgetfulness. The moderate and severe stages of the disease exhibit impaired concentration, comprehension and formulation of responses. In the last stages of the disease, muttering, groaning, grunting and moaning are the only means left in communication.

Managing communication is never an easy task in Alzheimer's disease. It involves the entire healthcare team. Lapses in memory render it difficult for family members to be easily recognized. There will be more confusion if members of the healthcare team keep changing frequently. Familiarity with faces is important in establishing trust.

Techniques of Communicating With the Diagnosed Person

Always treat the diagnosed person with dignity and as an adult person. Talk to them at eye level and always introduce new faces. Maintain eye contact at all times and show objects or point directions to augment what is being said. Eliminate environmental noise by turning off radios and televisions. Speak slowly and use short and familiar words. Do not use baby talk language, jargons, long statements and demeaning facial expressions. Praise achievements and completed tasks. Identify feelings and respond accordingly. Explain what is going to be done such as in transferring and bathing. Use simple questions that can be answered by a yes and a no. Allow sufficient time for responses. Provide a word if the person get stuck or is struggling for a word to use. Listen actively and carefully to avoid misinterpretation. Research has shown that people with the Alzheimer's disease respond well to non-verbal cues such as a smiling face, a gentle touch and a friendly tone of voice.

Chapter 9 — Managing the Activities of Daily Living

The different ADLs (activities of daily living) are eating, bathing, toileting, dressing and walking. Instrumental activities of daily living will include cooking and household work, shopping, telephoning, financial management and transportation. Changes and pattern in performing ADLs depends on the stages of the Alzheimer's disease and the over all functionality of the person.

Managing Eating

In the early stage of the disease, food preparation is minimal and self-feeding is automatic. The assistance that would be needed is preparing food such as cutting meat and pouring liquids. However, in the late stages, dependency on the caregiver and family members is a common scenario during mealtime. It is best to assess the nutritional needs of the diagnosed person. Prepare meals that are condensed in nutritional value containing protein, carbohydrates, essential fats, vitamins and minerals.

Meals should be regularly served at the same time in the same place. The diagnosed person should be assisted with hand washing if unable to do so. The mouth should be clean and the dentures should be worn. Make sure that dentures are in good condition to avoid aspiration. Avoid serving many foods because it is confusing. Older adults generally eat less. Do not use plastic utensils because they can break at anytime. Debone meat properly and cut into smaller pieces when serving food during the last stages of the disease.

Managing Bathing and Personal Hygiene

It is a challenge to motivate the diagnosed person to take a shower. It is a private activity requiring a lot of movement. Always set a regular time for bathing. Prepare and gather all necessary equipments. Use hypoallergenic soap if necessary. It would be best to walk with the person all the way to the bathroom before telling him about bathing because sometimes they refuse. If the person refuses; avoid force but wait for a while and try again. Adjust the temperature of the bathroom to make the person feel comfortable. Test the temperature of the water together. Use simple commands. Enable the person to participate in bathing by handing him the soap. Use a shower bench to avoid fatigue. Check the skin for wounds and lesions. Pat the skin to dry. Hand the towel if the person is able to dry himself. It is essential to provide assistive devices in the bathroom such as grab bars, hand held showers and benches. Offer a sponge bath if showering is not possible. Provide distraction and music if the person becomes agitated.

Oral hygiene can be a complex activity during the third to last stages of the disease. Brushing the teeth at least twice a day is a common practice. The diagnosed person may not be able to open toothpaste or to apply the paste on the toothbrush. Forgetting to spit the toothpaste and rinse the mouth can occur. Always inspect dentures for condition and fit. Assess the mouth for swollen gums and tooth decay. Assist in brushing teeth and gargling. Use electric razor for shaving the beard and moustache.

Managing Toilet and Elimination

The ability to use the toilet for elimination during the last stages of the disease is lost. There is total dependence. Incontinence commonly occurs during this stage. Urinary incontinence is the involuntary leakage of urine due to certain medications such as diuretics and narcotics. It is also caused by urinary tract infection, immobilization, enlarge prostate, incompetent urinary system and among others.

The most common urinary incontinences are stress, functional, overflow and urge. Stress incontinence is due to the inability of the bladder and urethra to withstand the amount of pressure from the urine. It occurs when a person is laughing, sneezing, coughing and lifting an object. Functional incontinence is due to inability or unwillingness of a person to use the toilet. This is the case when a person is immobile. Overflow incontinence is due to a full bladder. It occurs to persons with spinal cord injuries and bladder diseases. Urge incontinence is due to abnormal contractions of the urinary bladder. It occurs in diseases of the central nervous system.

Managing urinary incontinence requires a thorough assessment to determine the cause. Interventions can be implemented after determining the cause. Bladder retraining, pelvic exercises and biofeedback are interventions for the cognitively competent person. The person with Alzheimer's disease has a more simple approach. Provide emotional reassurance. Always provide privacy. Frequently encourage the person to use the toilet. Schedule the toilet usage on a regular basis. Consider the accessibility to the toilet. Provide a bedside commode if ambulation is not possible. Choose clothes that are easily removed. Provide verbal cues to enable the person to identify the bathroom. Provide incontinence pad and diapers. Stimulate urination by running water in the sink.

Managing Dressing

Dressing is a complicated task for a person with Alzheimer's disease. It requires motor skills, balancing and sequencing. All of these functions have deteriorated during the severe to last stages of the disease. Always provide privacy. All clothing equipment should be prepared. Remove all dirty clothes and put in laundry basket. The choices of clothes to wear should be simplified. Offer at least two different clothes. Clothes should be loose and with Velcro straps. Zippers and buttons are complicated for the diagnosed person. Hand the clothes one at a time. Give simple and direct instructions. Keep it organized. Start with underwear, then with the shirt and so on. Provide non-skid shoes.

Managing Ambulation and Walking

Walking is known to be the best exercise because it uses the different muscles of the body and promotes blood circulation. The ability to walk and to be mobile is lost during the last stages of the disease. It is important to maintain optimal functionality of the body. Avoid using a walker or cane because cognitive impairment will not allow the person to use these devices safely. Transfer and assistance is needed at all times. Consult with a physical therapist regarding muscle exercises. Take the person for a walk in the garden or in the park in the early stages of the disease.

Managing Activities

Majority of the instrumental activities of daily will be gone during the moderate to severe stages of the disease. Providing activities is helpful in enhancing the self-esteem and emotional well being of the diagnosed person. It stimulates mental activity and promotes physical exercises. It is also a means of distraction from behavioral symptoms. These activities should be voluntary, purpose driven and not competitive. Keep it simple and accomplish it in a short period of time. Activities should be directly related to the ability and skill of the person. Consider past hobbies and accomplishments. Always praise the diagnosed person after the activity. Do not criticize for mistakes. Always engage in conversation and encourage the person to express himself. Maintain safety at all times. Avoid sharp pointed objects such as scissors and cutters. Provide rest periods.

Art, crafts, music, gardening, community outing, picnics and recreation are excellent activities. Any activity outside the house promotes a sense of connection to the outside world. It enables the person to reminisce and recall happy memories.

Chapter 10 — Basic Home Care Management

The goal of disease management is basically to facilitate human action to achieve goals. Planning is one of the steps involved. It is also the most crucial step because it requires analyses from the information collected. Organizing comes after planning. To effectively organize a plan, it should involve the diseased person, caregivers, member of the household and healthcare professionals. Implement all these plans and give direction if it is necessary. Results occur after implementing the plans. This is a good time to gauge whether goals and expectations are met or revisions are needed. The cycle is repeated. Flexibility is of the essence.

Managing home care is a big challenge for all the members of the family. It is usually discussed after a diagnosis of Alzheimer's disease is confirmed. There are many things that are to be considered in managing the home care of the diagnosed member of the family. It should be flexible and in accordance with the current stage of the disease. Guidance and counseling is needed at all times.

A big part of management is data gathering. It is a necessity to get all the important information regarding home care from the physician and healthcare professionals such as nurses, social workers, dietician and physical therapists. Establish a baseline contact by getting all their telephone numbers. Organize a journal for doctor's appointment, visiting nurse's schedule and physical therapy sessions. Gather information about coexisting conditions, prescribed medication, healthcare coverage and community resources. Make a list of the different instructions that they gave. Ask questions and write down the answers. Emergency numbers should be listed and easily accessible to all caregivers and family members.

Gather all the important financial documents from the diagnosed person such as bank accounts, pension benefits, social security payments, mortgages, insurance policies and investment accounts. This information will be needed for future transactions in all aspects of the person's life. The family members should manage financial obligations of the diagnosed person. Arrange for benefit claims and pensions. Prepare tax returns, especially if there are ongoing investments. Pay the bills of mortgages, utilities, credit card purchases and loans. Pensions, disability checks and retirement accounts can be utilized to pay some of the home care expenditures.

Consider environmental changes at home. Set a bedroom that is near the bathroom for ease of access during incontinence. The bedroom should be far from the main door to avoid an escape during episodes of wandering. Lock the windows at all times. Ensure there are locks and alarm systems throughout the house. Put a bracelet on the diagnosed person's arm with his name and address just in case he or she escapes. Block the entrance to the second floor where there won't be anybody to supervise and monitor the diagnosed person. Remove any clutter such as throw rugs and electrical cords along pathways to prevent fall incidents. Put a nightlight in hallways. Simplify the house by decreasing the number of objects that are displayed. Use basic colors and simple choices to prevent confusion. Lock other rooms to prevent pillaging and hoarding. Place assistive devices in the bathroom such as grab bars, a hand held shower and a shower bench. All supplies relevant to home care such as personal care should be adequate.

Set up a schedule for a family member who will take care of the diagnosed person. Make shift changes depending on the stage of the disease to avoid role strain on the part of the family member. It is important to consider the job situation and availability of the family member. Hire a caregiver for respite care. Provide all the necessary instructions to the caregiver regarding meal preparation, bathing, grooming and toileting. Make sure to constantly check the physical condition of the diagnosed person. Take note of changes and consult the physician immediately.

Healthcare insurance coverage needs to be planned. The rising cost of healthcare will increase the monthly premiums. Private insurance will cover the majority of the home care but it also depends on the type of policy. Part A of Medicare will cover hospice care during the last stage of the disease for as long as there is a determination from the doctor. Part A also covers inpatient hospital care, some of the doctor fees and durable medical equipment. Part D of Medicare covers majority of the drugs that are prescribed by the doctor.

Establish advance directives in the early stages of the disease. It should include a living will and a durable power of attorney. These documents are done while the diagnosed person has some mental competence to express his end of life desires as well as the ability to sign them. The family members should decide who will act as the alternate decision maker if the diseased person is not mentally incompetent.

Attend a support group. Join different organizations that provide information and support for Alzheimer's disease. Conduct a research regarding community resources that can be use in coping with the disease. Reach out to friends and existing social networks.

References

I would like to express my gratitude to:

Dr. Lee Robbins for his support in writing this book.
Rich Grzesiak for editing this book.

Anatomy and Physiology, Wiley and Sons, New Jersey, 2007
Fundamentals of Nursing 7th Edition, Mosby, Canada, 2009
Gerontological Nursing 2nd Edition, ANCC, Maryland, 2009
Medical – Surgical Nursing 4th Edition, Prentice Hall, New Jersey, 2008
NCLEX PN, Saunders, Missouri, 2003
NCLEX RN, Mosby, Missouri, 1999
Nursing Assistants, Mosby, Philadelphia, 2004
Nursing Interventions and Clinical Skills, Mosby, Missouri, 2004
Nursing Procedures and Protocols, Lippincott, Philadelphia 2003
Pathophysiology of Disease 2nd Edition, Appleton and Lange, 1997
Pharmacology in Nursing 21st Edition, Mosby, Missouri 2001
Principles and Practice of Psychiatric Nursing 6th edition, Mosby, Missouri 1998
The Johns Hopkins Consumer Guide to Medical Tests, Medletter Associates Inc, New York, 2001
The Johns Hopkins White Papers, Hypertension and Stroke, Medletter Associates Inc, New York, 2003
Wikipidea Free Internet Dictionary

*** Book cover courtesy of Dr. Lee Robbins

Index

acetylcholine, 12, 21
activities of daily living, 6, 15, 16, 29
advance directives, 6, 33
age of senility, 9
aggression, 6, 25
aggressive behavior, 25, 26
agitated behavior, 25
agitation, 6, 21, 22, 24, 25, 26
agnosia, 15
agranulocytosis, 23
akathisia, 22
Aloysius Alzheimer, 9
Alzheimer's disease, 5, 6, 9, 11, 13, 14, 15, 16, 17, 18, 19, 21, 22, 24, 25, 26, 28, 29, 30, 32, 33
ambulating, 16
Amitriptyline (Elavil), 22
amyloid precursor protein, 11, 12
Antidepressants, 7, 22
anxiolytic (anti anxiety), 22
anxious, 22
aphasia, 15
ApoE4 (apolipoprotein), 11
APP (amyloid precursor protein), 11
apraxia, 15
arguing or disagreeing, 26
Aricept, 21
Aspiration, 19
assessment, 5, 9, 16, 24, 26, 30
assistance, 22, 23, 29, 31
assistive devices, 16, 29, 33
attention and language, 18
auditory hallucination, 26
Axis 3, 10
axon, 12
bathing, 6, 16, 28, 29, 33
bedside commode, 25, 30
benzodiazepines, 22
beta amyloid, 12
biofeedback, 30
bladder control, 15
bladder incontinence, 15
Bladder retraining, 30
Blocking, 7, 19

Blocking and Guarding Power Sources, 19
brain, 5, 6, 9, 11, 12, 13, 14, 15, 17, 18, 21, 22, 28
Bupropion (Wellbutrin), 22
carbon monoxide detectors, 16
caregiver, 6, 15, 19, 21, 24, 29, 33
central nervous system, 11, 21, 30
cerebellum, 18
cerebral cortex, 12, 13, 14
ChEIs (Cholinesterase inhibitors), 21
Chlordiaxepoxide (Librium), 22
Chlorpromazine (Thorazine), 22
circadian rhythm, 15
Citalopram (Celexa), 22
Classifying Alzheimer's disease, 10
clear pathways, 20
Clonazepam (Klonopin), 22
co morbidity, 11, 16
coccyx, 12
cognitive impairment, 19, 20, 31
Compliance, 21
confusion, 14, 21, 22, 25, 28, 33
constant moaning, 15
coping abilities, 15, 16
Cranial nerves, 18
CT (computed tomography), 17
cure, 13, 21
data gathering, 32
deep tendon reflexes, 18
dehydration, 24
delusion, 6, 22, 26
Delusion of grandeur, 26
delusion of persecution, 26
delusions, 10, 15, 26
dementia, 9, 10
dendrite, 12
dendrites, 12
diabetes, 4
diapers, 30
Diazepam (Valium), 22
difficulty in language, 15
difficulty in swallowing, 15, 19
disorientation, 9

dizziness, 17, 21
Donepizil (Aricept), 21
Dosage, 21, 22
dressing, 6, 15, 16, 29
drowsiness, 21, 22
Dry mouth, 22
DSM IV (Diagnostic and Statistical Manual of Mental Disorders), 10
Duloxetine (Cymbalta), 22
eating, 6, 16, 29
Emergency numbers, 32
emergency response system, 16
emotional reassurance, 30
environmental changes, 32
Environmental hazards, 17
Enzymes, 12
Escitalopram (Lexapro), 22
Exelon, 21
fall risk factors, 17
family dynamics, 16
family member, 16, 33
feelings about self, 16
feelings of hopelessness, 27
financial documents, 32
financial obligations, 32
Fluoxetine (Prozac), 22
Folstein test, 17
food preparation, 29
forgetfulness, 28
forgets, 15
forgetting, 14
Friedrich Lewy, 10
frontal lobe, 12, 13
Functional incontinence, 30
Galantamine (Razadyne), 21
gastrointestinal discomfort, 21
glutamate receptor, 21
grab bars, 29, 33
guarding, 19
Guidance and counseling, 19, 32
hallucination, 6, 22, 26
hallucinations, 15, 26
hand held showers, 29
health care insurance, 18
healthcare professionals, 32
hippocampus, 12, 13, 14
history, 14, 15, 16, 26
Hoarding behavior, 25
Home care, 19
home environment, 16
hospice care, 33
Hospice care, 15
household member, 16, 24
hyperthermia, 19
hypothermia, 19
impaired, 16, 19, 21, 27, 28
impaired cognition, 19
impulse control, 19
inability to rationalize, 19
inability to recall, 14
inability to stay still, 22
incontinence, 24, 30, 32
incontinence pad, 30
insoluble plaque, 12
insomnia, 22
Installing Devices to Prevent Leaving the House, 7, 20
installing locks and alarm systems, 24
instrumental activities of daily living, 16
insurance coverage, 6, 33
interpretation of sensation, 12
interview, 16, 18
irritability, 15
judgment and reasoning, 17
laboratory tests, 5, 18
language and comprehension, 17
language competence, 17
Lewy bodies, 9
Life review, 27
lightheadedness, 22
Lorazepam (Ativan), 22
loss of ability, 15
loss of impulse control, 15
low self-esteem, 27
lumbar vertebrae, 12
Managing Activities, 8, 31
Managing Ambulation and Walking, 8, 31
Managing Bathing and Personal Hygiene, 8, 29
Managing Dressing, 8, 30
Managing Eating, 8, 29

Managing Toilet and Elimination, 8, 30
medical conditions, 16
Medicare, 33
medications, 5, 19, 21, 22, 23, 30
Memantine (Namenda), 21
memory and recall, 17
memory loss, 9, 14, 16
mental exercises, 11
mental status, 17
mental tests, 5, 17
microtubules, 12
Mirtazapine (Remeron), 22
Misdiagnosis, 9
misplacing, 14
MMSE (Mini Mental State Examination), 17
monoamine oxidase inhibitor (MAOI), 22
Motor neurons, 12
motor problems, 15
MRI (magnetic resonance imaging), 17
multi infarct dementia, 9
Namenda, 21
nerve cells, 12, 21
Neuroleptics, 7, 22
neurological examination, 5, 18
Neurons, 12
neuropathology, 9
neurotransmitter, 21
neurotransmitters, 12, 22
nightlight, 32
NMDA (N Methyl D Aspartate), 21
NMDA glutamate receptors, 21
non-skid shoes, 20, 30
non-verbal cues, 28
norepinephrine, 22
nucleus, 12
nutritional needs, 29
obeying a command, 17
occipital lobe, 12
Olanzapine (Zyprexa), 22
orientation, 11, 17
orientation to time and place, 17
orthostatic hypotension, 17
over the counter medications, 16
Overflow incontinence, 30
overmedication, 19
packet of questions, 16
parietal lobe, 12
Parkinson's disease, 18
pelvic exercises, 30
pesticides, 11
PET (positron emission tomography), 17
Pharmacology, 34
physician, 16, 17, 18, 21, 22, 24, 26, 32, 33
pill boxes, 21
Pillaging behavior, 25
plaques, 5, 9, 11, 13, 14, 15, 21, 22
praise, 31
Pre senile dementia, 9
Preventing Fall Accidents, 7, 20
privacy, 30
Prochlorperazine (Compazine), 22
Promethazine (Phenergan), 22
PSI (presenilin), 11
psychological history, 16
purposeful wandering behavior, 24
Quetiapine (Seroquel), 22
Razadyne, 21
recall, 15, 31
recreational drug, 16
registering names of objects, 17
remember, 14
Reminiscing, 27
Removal of Objects that Can Cause Physical Injuries, 7, 19
Reorientation, 21
repetition skills, 17
Repetitive behavior, 15
repetitive fashion, 15
restless behavior, 25
retain information, 15
rigidity, 23
Risperidone (Risperdal), 22
Rivastigmine (Exelon), 21
Rummaging behavior, 25
sacrum, 12
safety, 5, 6, 14, 16, 19, 21, 31
selective serotonin reuptake inhibitor (SSRI), 22
self esteem, 27

self-care, 15, 24
self-esteem, 31
sensory deficits, 17
Sensory neurons, 12
serotonin, 22
Sertraline (Zoloft), 22
Shadowing, 8, 24
shadowing behavior, 24
shingles virus, 11
side effects, 16, 21, 22, 23, 25
signs and symptoms, 18, 21
silver staining technique, 9
simple commands, 29
social networking, 11
social support, 16
Somatic hallucinations, 26
sound stimulus, 12
Spinal nerves, 12
store memories, 12
Stress incontinence, 30
stress level, 16
sundowning behavior, 25
supervision, 21, 23
suspiciousness, 15
synapse, 12

Tacrine, 21
tangles, 5, 9, 11, 12, 13, 14, 15, 21, 22
tardive dyskinesia, 22
tau protein, 12
tearfulness, 15
temporal lobe, 12
Thioridazine (Mellaril), 22
toilet usage, 30
toileting, 6, 15, 16, 29, 33
total dependence, 15, 30
toxins, 11
tremors, 23
tricyclic antidepressant (TCA), 22
trigger factor, 24, 25, 26
Urge incontinence, 30
Vascular dementia, 9
violence, 26
Visual interpretation, 12
vulgar language, 15
wandering, 6, 15, 24, 32
Wandering, 8, 20, 24
wandering behavior, 24
Wandering behavior, 20
withdrawal, 23, 24
write a sentence, 17

***Kindly write a review about this book for Amazon or other sites to help other readers that could benefit from this text. Thank you.

And please feel free to browse my other books @ Amazon.com

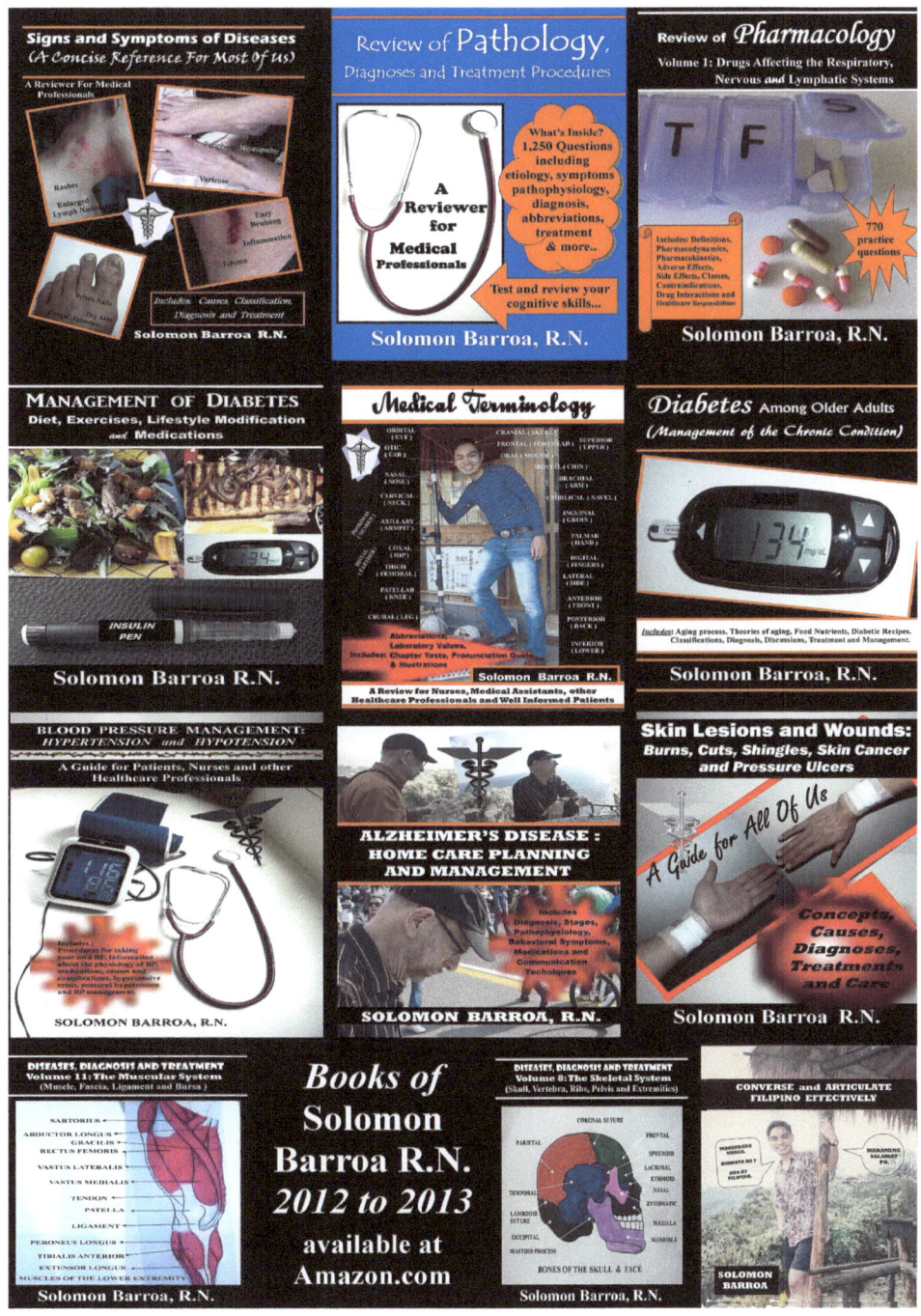

Connect with me online :

Facebook: http://www.facebook.com/solomon.barroa
Twitter: https://twitter.com/solomonbarroa
Amazon: amazon.com/author/solomonbarroa
LinkedIn: http://www.linkedin.com/in/solomonbarroa

www.ingramcontent.com/pod-product-compliance
Lightning Source LLC
Chambersburg PA
CBHW050354180526
45159CB00005B/2008